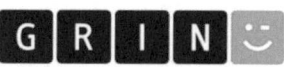

Bibliographic information published by the German National Library:

The German National Library lists this publication in the National Bibliography; detailed bibliographic data are available on the Internet at http://dnb.dnb.de .

Imprint:

Copyright © 2016 GRIN Verlag, Open Publishing GmbH
Print and binding: Books on Demand GmbH, Norderstedt Germany
ISBN: 9783656986553

This book at GRIN:

http://www.grin.com/en/e-book/334786/drug-testing-and-volunteer-work-should-be-mandatory-for-welfare-recipients

Hassan Nawaz

Drug testing and volunteer work should be mandatory for welfare recipients

GRIN Publishing

GRIN - Your knowledge has value

Since its foundation in 1998, GRIN has specialized in publishing academic texts by students, college teachers and other academics as e-book and printed book. The website www.grin.com is an ideal platform for presenting term papers, final papers, scientific essays, dissertations and specialist books.

Visit us on the internet:

http://www.grin.com/

http://www.facebook.com/grincom

http://www.twitter.com/grin_com

Should drug testing and volunteer work be mandatory for welfare recipients?

1.	Introduction	2
1.1	Problem statement	2
1.2	Objectives of the research	2
1.3	Research questions	3
1.4	Thesis statement	3
2.	Literature review	3
2.1	Legislative proposals by different states:	4
2.2	Legislative proposals lead to legislative enactments:	4
3.	Favor or not to favor the drug testing and volunteer work:	5
4.	Does drug testing welfare really works?	5
5.	Statistics about the drug abuses and cost involved in ThinkProgress:	6
6.	Ethics involved in testing drugs	11
7.	Conclusion and the Future of Drug Testing	11
	References	12

1. Introduction

Substance abuse has always remained an issue for the policy makers and public assistance. States have proposed to test drugs presence in the recipients who have been benefiting from the public welfare, since 1996's federal welfare reform. Federal rules have allowed to test the presence of drugs as the part of Temporary Assistance for the Needy Families Blocks. Recently, almost all of the states have proposed drug screening and testing amongst the applicants. Through the public assistance programs of 2009, almost 20 states have proposed their legislation and have shown the requirement of drug testing as the eligibility criteria. However, the proposals could not become law due to the reason that legislation was based over random or suspicious drug testing. Now the need is to make drug testing mandatory so that government can save lots of money, provided as the public assistance to the non-deserving families, (Guthrie, 2010).

2011 sessions have brought new momentum in the proposal. After that, almost 12 states have passed their legislation and enacted it as a law. It is also important for the remaining states to go for the drug screening and measure the requirement of TANF for the illegal use of the drugs.

1.1   Problem statement

US government has passed almost $11.0 billion in supporting the drug welfare families, educating them and preventing diseases in them. It is no doubt a huge amount to be allocated in the budget of 2016, (National Drug Control Budget, 2015). It is no doubt a sympathetic situation that government is spending so much for saving the drug victims and compromising the other important areas of infrastructure development, education, health care, etc. Plus, the taxes paid by the taxpayers are also wasting due to this. It is a matter of great consideration that drug testing and the work of volunteers should be made mandatory to test the presences of drugs in recipient, before allowing them to enjoy aid.

1.2   Objectives of the research

- To examine the long and short term benefits of making drug testing and volunteer work mandatory
- To evaluate the ethical dilemma for the drug welfare recipients
- To gauge the statistical figures for the federal governments who have made drug testing mandatory

1.3   Research questions

What are the benefits derived from making drug testing and volunteer work mandatory?

1.4   Thesis statement

Many of the states have passed their legislation and enacted drug testing as a law. They have attained positive outcomes while stopping aiding un-needy families. In this analytical work, the idea behind the drug testing and volunteer work will be analyzed, (Budd, 2010). The supporting and opposing views will be examined with the ethical dilemma for the drug aid recipients. Plus, the statistical analysis will be done for the states that have incorporated drug test and volunteer work mandatory. And benefits for the federal governments will be evaluated for the drug testing welfare.

2.   Literature review

Drug abuses are very common in the US. US government has announced the federal funds for supporting the families of drug addicts and to save them from becoming victim. However, almost 8,300 people died due to the abuse of drugs, in the year 2003. Through 1999, there is increment of almost 300% in drug victims and deaths. Government supporting programs are not working well and they have failed in stopping people to become victim. One of the reasons identified is the deficiency of the drug knowledge and results caused due to over doses of drugs. Many people have no idea that what are the consequences of taking extra dose of drugs and they become helpless later on, (Macdonald, Bois, Brands, Dempsey, Erickson, Marsh, & Chiu, 2011). Government has tough announced to support these families financially and giving their loved ones a better life. But what welfare recipients are doing? Need is to extract answer to this question.

Study done by Socha, (2001) has indicated that recipients of drugs welfare are spending most of the aided money on buying drugs. The researcher has pinpointed that large share of state's welfare is being given to support the drug victims so that they can have better life, yet their drug usage is losing benefits of the welfare.

2.1 Legislative proposals by different states:

On March 28, 2016, almost seventeen states have enacted the law for addressing substance abuse and testing of drug presences for the participation in the welfare program. On March 23, 2016, Governor Tomblin of West Virginia signed SB 6. SB 6 was a screening program for the drug welfare participants. When the caseworker finds the person as a drug abuser he will order for further drug testing. If the positive result extracted from testing drug by the volunteer workers than applicant is required to attend the substance abuse treatment, job development skills program and counseling. His or her family will continuously receive designated welfare amount. Those who have refused to undergo drug screening will consider being ineligible to get welfare assistance, (Guthrie, 2011).

2.2 Legislative proposals lead to legislative enactments:

Almost 18 states including Illinois, Kentucky, Minnesota, Connecticut, New York, West Virginia, Vermont, South Carolina, Oregon, Rhode Island, Virginia, Massachusetts, Montanan, Pennsylvania and Maine have proposed the need of drug testing and volunteer work. They have asked their state to study the highlighted issue and pass the bill. Even Missouri has also proposed the use of drug testing and volunteer work for SNAP or Supplemental Nutrition Assistance Program.

On April 8, 2015, Governor Hutchinson of Arkansas has signed the SB 600 and makes it as a law. It is declared to be mandatory to check and screen presence of drugs and based on drug testing applicant can go for TANF. The Department of the Workforce Services has been designated with the duty to establish two year pilot study over the drug welfare and volunteer work's program, (Macdonald, Bois, Brands, Dempsey, Erickson, Marsh, & Chiu, 2011). The Governor has also asked to execute the program over cities of Oklahoma, Tennessee, Missouri and Mississippi, (all of these states have already passed their drug testing and volunteer work laws).

In the budget bill of SB 21 of Wisconsin, it is advised to the participating individuals that they should go for drug test from the volunteer work. The program developed by Wisconsin Volunteer Work and Transform Milwaukee Jobs to train and educate the experience programs for the non-custodial parents. The bill also indicated the addition of test for the Supplement Nutrition Assistance Program SNAP so that employment training can only be given to the drug abusers.

3.   Favor or not to favor the drug testing and volunteer work:

According to the work of Kelly, (working in the Kansan House since 2005) has proposed the bill that there should be no spending done over drug welfare. However her bill was not passed in Senate. Kelly however believes that she and the other state sponsors of the drug testing bills should no way support the drug habits by paying dollars. She also argued that even keeping eye on the usage of public assistance would not even say money (Sulzberger, 2011).

On oppose, the work of Craig P. Blair passed in the house of West Virginia who has appreciated and respected the work of the taxpayers that are helping drug addicted in becoming work-qualified and good parents.

It is being criticized by many policy makers that the bill presented by Pollack, Danziger, Jayakody, & Seefeldt, (2012) was unconstitutional. It was already written in the welfare program that drug addicted person will be referred for screening or treatment. However, the favoring parties are more concerned for the helping and aiding the addicts and are not ready to leave them to die. They said volunteers and their jobs can be done in different manner. They can also serve in guiding and helping drug addicts from leaving their habit, rather than dehumanizing by testing or screening them.

4.   Does drug testing welfare really works?

There are very few benefits encountered through drug testing and volunteer work program. It is obtained that the claims made by states that drug testing and volunteer work programs will save them money was absolutely wrong. They found that it was quite easy and cheap to help the drug addicts for rooting out their drug addiction. But it is completely false as the cost of treatment is so high that states cannot really afford. Moreover, the case markers believe that funds allocated for the welfare if not going for the TANF program, still it is going for the drug testing. So, it is far better to help child of the drug addicts and provide them cash assistance rather than providing extra money to the administrative pots, (Socha, 2001).

Another reason for not supporting the drug testing and volunteer work mentioned by them is the increasing stigma around the drug use and the welfare. Drug testing enhances shame in the people and they feel shy to ask for the welfare, from the fear of test outcomes. People may not want to disclose their habit and may not want drug abuse treatment. It is also found

5

that people who are proofed to be drug addict and needs to avail treatment; may have to wait long for the attainment of treatment because of the long awaited lines, (Carey, 2008).

On the other side, drug test and volunteer work favoring party feel that if government make drug test mandatory, no undeserving families will claim welfare. Though initial cost of the programs and drug testing is expensive; but in the long term it will eradicate the cruse of drug and will also help the entire family from getting out of the drug curse. Treatment is no doubt expensive but it will make a person to avail benefit in the long run. Entire family will reap out benefit and society will become a better place to live in.

In this regards, government of many states have made collaborated efforts in starting the ThinkProgress project. In this project, it is assured that only those victims of drug will be supported who have passed their drug test and have shown willingness to go for the treatment. The outcomes of this project has started showing up. Although it is found that in starting the rewards are extremely low and cost is extremely high, but it will have real impact on the future of entire US, (Jayakody, Danziger, & Pollack, 2010).

5.   Statistics about the drug abuses and cost involved in ThinkProgress:

Initial outcomes of the ThinkProgress test have shown ineffective outcomes in different states. It is found that in Missouri, there were drug testing and volunteer work initiated in 2011 and it has provided the evidence in March 2014 that there were 38970 participants who were tested and only 48 found to be positive drug abusers. The total budget allocated for the single project was about $336,297. It was said by the spokeswoman of Department of the Social Services, that the initial cost for the three year program is about $1.35 million. The graph is presented below as:

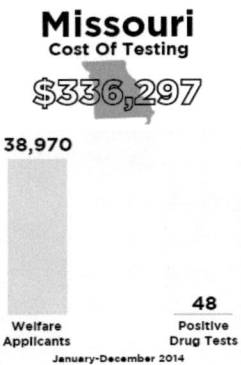

Missouri
Cost Of Testing

$336,297

38,970

48

Welfare
Applicants

Positive
Drug Tests

January-December 2014

Source: ThinkProgress Org., (2015)

In the state of Oklahoma, there were drug testing and volunteer work initiated in 2012 and it has provided the evidence in November 2014 that there were 3342 participants who were tested and only 2992 selected for the further testing. Out of 2992, only 297 were found to be drug abusers. The total budget allocated for the single project was about $385,872. It was said by the spokesman of Department of the Human Services, that the initial cost for the 2013-2014 year program is about $185,219. The graph is presented below as:

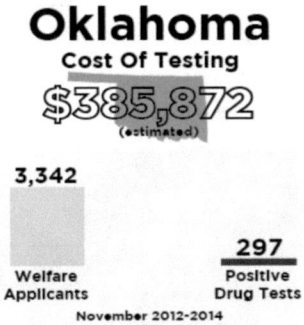

Oklahoma
Cost Of Testing

$385,872
(estimated)

3,342

297

Welfare
Applicants

Positive
Drug Tests

November 2012-2014

Source: ThinkProgress Org., (2015)

In the state of Utah, there were drug testing and volunteer work initiated in 2012 and it has provided the evidence in July 2014. The test was announced to be written screening followed with the drug test, (Gov., 2016). 9552 participants were screened and out of them only 838 were taken for the drug test. Out of 838, only 29 were found to be drug abusers. The total budget allocated for the single project was about $64,000. It was said by the spokesman of Department of the Human Services, that the initial cost for two years program is about $64,566. The graph is presented below as:

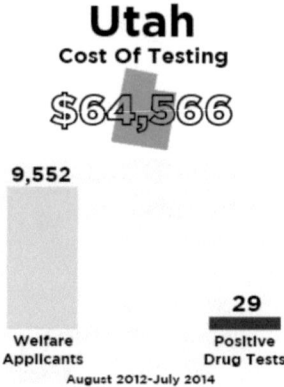

Source: ThinkProgress Org., (2015)

In the state of Kansas, there were drug testing and volunteer work initiated in 2013 and it has provided the evidence in 2014 that there were 2783 participants for the TANF who were tested and only 11 individuals were found to be drug abusers. The total budget allocated for the single project was about $40,000. It was said by the spokeswoman of Kansas Department of the Children and Families, that the initial cost for the six months program is about $40,000. The graph is presented below as:

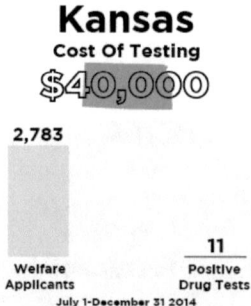

Source: ThinkProgress Org., (2015)

In the state of Mississippi, there were written questionnaire about the use of drug and mandatory drug test later on. It has provided the evidence in August 2014 that there were 3656 participants for the TANF who were tested and only 38 were referred for drug testing. Only 2 appear to be positive drug abusers out of 38. The total budget allocated for the single project was about $5290. It was said by the spokeswoman of Mississippi Department of the Human Services, that the initial cost for the six months program is about $5290. The graph is presented below as:

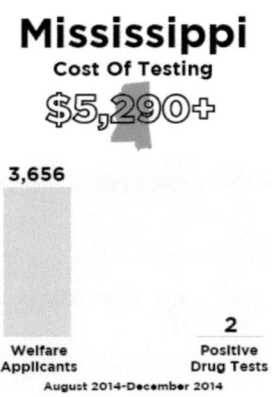

Mississippi
Cost Of Testing
$5,290+

3,656

2

Welfare
Applicants

Positive
Drug Tests

August 2014-December 2014

Source: ThinkProgress Org., (2015)

In the state of Tennessee, there were drug testing and volunteer work initiated in 2012 and it has provided the evidence in July 2014 that there were 16017 participants for the TANF who were tested and only 37 individuals were found to be drug abusers. The total budget allocated for the single project was about $5295. It was said by the spokesman of Tennessee Department of the Human Services, that the initial cost for the first fiscal year program is about $5295. The graph is presented below as:

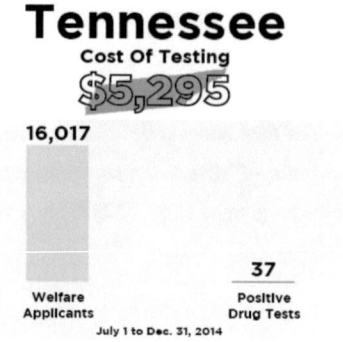

Tennessee
Cost Of Testing
$5,295

16,017

Welfare
Applicants

37
Positive
Drug Tests

July 1 to Dec. 31, 2014

Source: ThinkProgress Org., (2015)

In the state of Arizona, there were drug testing and volunteer work initiated in 2009 and it has provided the evidence in July 2014 that there were 142,424 participants for the TANF who were tested and only 3 individuals were found to be drug abusers. The total budget allocated for the single project was about $499. It was said by the spokesman of Arizona Department of the Economic Security, that the initial cost for the first fiscal year program is about $1.7 million. The graph is presented below as:

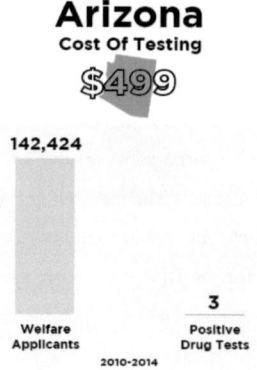

Arizona
Cost Of Testing
$499

142,424

Welfare
Applicants

3
Positive
Drug Tests

2010-2014

Source: ThinkProgress Org., (2015)

6. Ethics involved in testing drugs

Ethically it is said that it is not advisable to go for the drug testing. The reason for not supporting the drug testing and volunteer work mentioned by Jayakody, Danziger, & Pollack, (2010) is the increasing stigma around the drug use and the welfare. Drug testing enhances shame in the people and they feel shy to ask for the welfare, from the fear of test outcomes. People may not want to disclose their habit and may not want drug abuse treatment. In this case many families will remain in miserable condition.

7. Conclusion and the Future of Drug Testing

It is explored that US government has passed almost $11.0 billion in supporting the drug welfare families, educating them and preventing diseases in them. It is no doubt a huge amount to be allocated in the budget of 2016, (National Drug Control Budget, 2015). It is no doubt a sympathetic situation that government is spending so much for saving the drug victims and compromising the other important areas of infrastructure development, education, health care, etc. Further it is explored that drug abuses are very common in the US. US government has announced the federal funds for supporting the families of drug addicts and to save them from becoming victim. However, almost 8,300 people died due to the abuse of drugs, in the year 2003.

Some proposed that there should be no spending done over drug welfare. There should be no way support the drug habits by paying dollars. They have argued that even keeping eye on the usage of public assistance would not even say money. On oppose, some has appreciated and respected the work of the taxpayers that are helping drug addicted in becoming work-qualified and good parents.

It is found that drug test and volunteer work favoring party feel that if government make drug test mandatory, no undeserving families will claim welfare. Though initial cost of the programs and drug testing is expensive; but in the long term it will eradicate the cruse of drug and will also help the entire family from getting out of the drug curse. Treatment is no doubt expensive but it will make a person to avail benefit in the long run.

References

Budd, J. C. (2010). Pledge your body for your bread: Welfare, drug testing, and the inferior fourth amendment. *Wm. & Mary Bill Rts. J., 19*, 751.

Carey, C. A. (2008). Crafting a challenge to the practice of drug testing welfare recipients: federal welfare reform and state response as the most recent chapter in the war on drugs. *Buff. L. Rev., 46*, 281.

Gov., (2016). Fy16 Budget highlights. *Online.* Accessed on 16th April 2016. Available at <https://www.whitehouse.gov///sites/default/files/ondcp/press-releases/ondcp_fy16_budget_highlights.pdf>

Guthrie, P. M. (2010). Drug Testing and Welfare: Taking the Drug War to Unconstitutional Limits. *Ind. LJ, 66*, 579.

Jayakody, R., Danziger, S., & Pollack, H. (2010). Welfare reform, substance use, and mental health. *Journal of Health Politics, Policy and Law, 25*(4), 623-652.

Macdonald, S., Bois, C., Brands, B., Dempsey, D., Erickson, P., Marsh, D., ... & Chiu, A. (2011). Drug testing and mandatory treatment for welfare recipients. *International Journal of Drug Policy, 12*(3), 249-257.

Pollack, H. A., Danziger, S., Jayakody, R., & Seefeldt, K. S. (2012). Drug testing welfare recipients—false positives, false negatives, unanticipated opportunities. *Women's Health Issues, 12*(1), 23-31.

Sulzberger, A. G. (2011). States adding drug test as hurdle for welfare. *New York Times, 10.*

Socha, M. D. (2001). Analysis of Michigan's Plan for Suspicionless Drug Testing of Welfare Recipients under the Fourth Amendment Special Needs Exception, An. *Wayne L. Rev., 47*, 1099.

ThinkProgress Org., (2015). Drug testing by state. *Online.* Accessed on 16th April 2016. Available at <http://thinkprogress.org/economy/2015/02/26/3624447/tanf-drug-testing-states/>

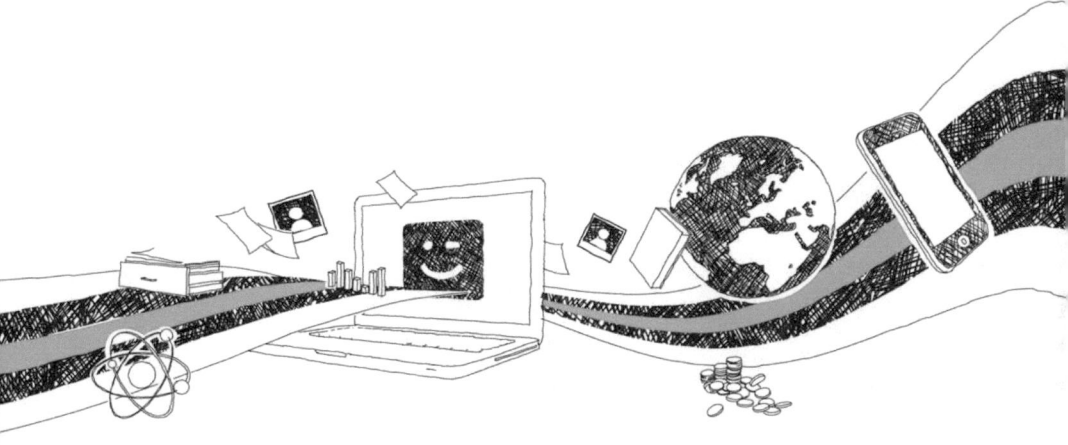
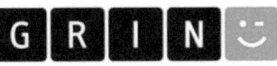